Fennel Essential Oil

Benefits, Properties, Applications, Studies & Recipes

by Ann Sullivan

Published in USA by:

Ann Sullivan
217 N. Seacrest Blvd #9
Boynton Beach
FL 33425

© Copyright 2017

ISBN-13: ISBN-13: 978-1546916178
ISBN-10: 1546916172

Table of Contents

Introduction 8

Chapter 1 – Benefits of Fennel Essential Oil...............13

  Cultivation of Fennel 13

  A History of Fennel..14

    Chemical Components 16

  Main Properties of Fennel Essential Oil..................16

    Antioxidant...17

    Antispasmodic 18

    Antiseptic...18

    Antiparasitic 18

    Antifungal...19

    Diuretic 19

    Expectorant...19

    Galactogogue 19

    Laxative..20

    Stimulant...20

    Carminative 20

    Emmenagogue 20

    Stomachic 21

    Tonic 21

  Common Therapeutic Uses 21

Cardiovascular Wellness 21

Cancer 22

Blood Pressure 22

Digestive Wellness 23

Immune System Booster 23

Women's Wellness 23

Eye Wellness 24

Respiratory Issues 24

Safety Precautions & Common Applications 25

Safety 25

Blends 26

Chapter 2 – Recipes for Fennel Essential Oil 27

Pure Applications 27

Anxiety 27

Blood Clots 28

Bruises 28

Courage 28

Detoxing 29

Digestive Aid 29

Flatulence 29

Gastritis 29

Hormone Balance 30

Intestinal Parasite 30

Kidney Stones 30

Lactation (Increase) 30

Liver Support 30

Menstrual Cramps 31

Motivation 31

Nausea 31

Pancreas Support 32

PMS 32

Prostate Support 32

Prostatic Hyperplasia (Benign Enlargement of the Prostate) 32

Skin Renewal 32

Stomach Cramps 33

Strength 33

Urinary Stones 33

Wrinkles 33

Blends 34

Anti-Wrinkle Solution 34

Constipation/Diarrhea 35

Courage Blend 36

Craving Crasher 37

Diuretic Bath 38

Gout 39

Hot Flash Relief...40

Indigestion..41

Lymphatic Support 42

Regulate Menstruation..43

Reproductive Wellness Salve.................................44

Stomach Cramps 45

Stress-Reducing Massage Oil................................46

Swollen Feet...47

Uplifting Blend 48

Water Retention..49

Chapter 3 – Fennel Essential Oil Studies 51

Study 1 – Anxiolytic Activity 51

Study 2 – Antimicrobial Properties.............................53

Study 3 – Antioxidant, Anti-inflammatory & Anti-proliferative Properties...55

Study 4 – Antifungal Properties 57

Study 5 – Antifungal Properties 59

Study 6 – Anticarcinogenic & Antioxidant Properties 61

Chapter 4 – The Ins & Outs of Essential Oils 63

Where do essential oils come from? 63

How are essential oils extracted?..............................64

Pressing Method..64

Distillation Method 64

Solvent Method 65

Maceration Method...65

How do you use essential oils? 66

Topical Administration..67

Inhalation Therapy..68

Ingestion 68

What are the general benefits of using essential oils?
....69

Replacement for Prescription Drugs.....................69

Cheap, but Effective Alternative 70

No Expiration Date 70

Versatility..70

Conclusion..72

Introduction

What are essential oils, and how might they be used for therapeutic purposes?

Essential oils are ultra-potent oils, extracted from plants and flowers that have been utilized in medicine for centuries. Presently, they're most commonly used to supplement pharmaceutical medication, but they can also be an effective alternative to pharmaceuticals if you don't have access to them. Before you dismiss essential oils to support the body's natural defenses against injuries and illness, look at the historical evidence of the oils' therapeutic competence in practice. Your average age-old medical text will demonstrate that essential oils, herbs, and plenty of other natural ingredients have, for thousands of years, successfully enhanced immune function to meet and defeat any number of ailments and injuries. Though traditional medicine is considered "alternative" now, it was once the gold standard. And, frankly, perhaps it still should be, as these natural age-tested remedies can fortify the body's battlements against everything from simple maladies, like headaches, cuts and bruises, to serious diseases, like cancer.

Essential oils are deemed "essential," because the oils are composed of the "essence" of the plant. The difference between essential oils and other oils – like olive oil or vegetable oil, for instance – is that essential oils have high volatility and reduced fixation, which results in faster evaporation, enabling their popular use in aromatherapy.

Even at high temperatures, olive and vegetable oils don't evaporate.

Essential oils are especially necessary when it comes to a major natural or man-made disaster or some potential viral outbreak. In these types of dire situations, you may not have quick access (or any access at all) to your standard pharmaceutical supply; so, essential oils, along with other alternative medicines, will be your go-to wellness aids in the case of social collapse, viral outbreak or devastating natural disaster. When medical access is null and void, alternatives to our modern-day standard are the only chance we have to keep pathogens at bay.

You probably don't realize that you already use essential oils every day. They're in perfumes, shampoos, soaps, ointments...they're even used in furniture polish. Why are they found in so many aromatic products? Well, basically, because essential oils are super concentrated aromatic liquids, so their scent is remarkably strong. Let's put this into perspective: to steam tea, you use a few leaves of peppermint or juniper; to produce a single ounce of essential oil, five whole *pounds* of peppermint or juniper leaves are required. Some sources claim that to produce twelve pounds of essential oil would necessitate an acre of peppermint, juniper, or any other oil you're looking to produce en masse. Unlike vegetable oil, you don't often find concentrated therapeutic-grade essential oils sold in bulk, instead the oils are often sold in easily carried small, dark bottles, perfect for your GOOD bag (Get Out Of Dodge). Which is exactly what this book is aiming to help you do –

get out of dodge with your most vital of essential oils intact, a good supply of fennel essential oil.

Why fennel, you ask? Well, to get you quickly up to speed on this most essential of oils, below we've provided a condensed synopsis of fennel, after which we'll outline in greater detail the oil's history, properties, and common therapeutic uses, so that you – the consumer – might have a better understanding of the oil's benefits and applications. We've even provided supportive remedies for pure fennel, as well as blended recipes that incorporate the valuable oil. Chapter 3 will further detail past scientific research on fennel essential oil.

Now, let's get down to it.

Essential Oil 101: the Basics of Fennel

Summary: Fennel, or Foeniculum vulgare, has been used since the days of ancient Egypt and Rome for both spiritual and therapeutic purposes. Warriors used fennel to enhance power, bravery and longevity in battle. Therapeuticly, it was used to support the body's defenses against everything from earaches to snake bites. It was also used to create balance in the female reproductive system. During the Middle Ages, fennel took on an even more powerful application: it served to defend against witches, evil spirits and harmful spells. Present day applications of fennel include use in culinary dishes, supporting digestive issues, strengthening the respiratory and circulatory systems, and restoring balance to the female reproductive system.

Description: Fennel oil is commonly extracted through steam distillation. The seed is most often used. The oil is clear yellow in color, thin in consistency, and has a somewhat strong sweet, licorice scent.

Uses: Beyond those applications previously mentioned, additional uses for fennel essential oil include supporting the body's defenses against nausea, flatulence, halitosis, bruises, cellulite, gums, mouth, obesity, digestive issues, toxin build-up, cramps, PMS, menopause, water retention and healthy circulatory, respiratory and glandular function. When it comes to mood and emotion, fennel oil can help boost confidence and restore balance and stability.

Properties: Antioxidant, antispasmodic, antiseptic, antiparasitic, antifungal, antitoxic, diuretic, expectorant, galactogogue, laxative, stimulant, and tonic.

Application: Use neat or undiluted. You can apply topically, inhale directly, diffuse or use as a dietary supplement.

Safety Precautions: Fennel has been approved by the FDA for internal consumption and so can be used as a dietary supplement. Fennel oil is a dermal sensitizer, so dilute heavily if you have sensitive skin. Do not take in large quantities or if pregnant or epileptic.

Fun facts: Fennel is so named, because it's derived from the Latin word for "hay," which is "fenum."

Fennel comes from the parsley family and had many

applications by the Ancient Romans, one being to clear up cloudy vision. Being as such, they called it the "herb of sight."

Chapter 1 – Benefits of Fennel Essential Oil

Fennel essential oil offers several therapeutic benefits; but you may be wondering what these benefits are. In this chapter, we'll take a closer look at the history of fennel and its many uses.

Cultivation of Fennel

Fennel, or Foeniculum vulgare, is a flowering plant and perennial herb belonging to the celery family. The plant is native to the Mediterranean, grows to be up to 2.5 meters tall, and produces delicate feathery leaves and yellow flowers. The leaves are quite like dill and grow to be 40 cm long on average, while the flowers appear in groupings of 20 to 50 per section. The plant produces a dry seed fruit which grows to be anywhere from 4 to 10 mm long. The seed is commonly used to produce fennel essential oil.

Fennel has been cultivated all over the world, particularly near rivers and the sea, as it thrives best in dry soil near water. It can now be found in the US, Canada, Australia, Asia, and Europe and is especially prevalent alongside roads and in open fields, so much so that it's considered an invasive species in some regions of America and Australia. With a taste like anise, fennel is very flavorful and strongly scented, which makes the plant a flavoring source for foods and other products. There are also different subspecies of fennel, such as F. vulgare var. azoricum, also known as "Florence fennel." This subspecies is milder and sweeter in flavor, smaller than wild fennel, and stronger in smell. Very similar to anise, it is often mislabeled as such in grocery chains in North America.

A History of Fennel

The name "fennel" is derived from the Latin word "fenum," which means "hay." The Old English believed fennel to be a charm, and it is one of the Anglo-Saxon's "Nine Herbs Charms," which were determined by the pagans in the 10th century.

Fennel has a variety of applications, one being in the making of absinthe. The Florence fennel subspecies is used in this alcohol, which originated in Switzerland and was originally branded as medicine before it became popular in other countries around the latter half of the 1800s.

All parts of fennel are used internationally in culinary dishes, including the seeds, the bulb, and the leaves. The seeds are best used in cooking when they're green and fresh. When they turn grey they lose their potency. They are often used to flavor sweets and other desserts. In Pakistan and India, fennel seeds are coated with sugar and used in mukwas, which is akin to an after-dinner mint to freshen the breath. Fennel seeds are also an ingredient in toothpaste and even certain types of herbal tea.

The plant's bulb can be eaten raw or cooked in several ways – sautéed, grilled, stewed, or steamed. The leaves are not as flavorful as the rest of the plant, but can be used to flavor soups, salads, and sauces, as well as to garnish. The plant's flowers carry the strongest flavor and are, therefore, the most expensive.

Middle Eastern countries, such as Iran, Afghanistan, Pakistan, and India, use fennel seeds frequently in culinary dishes and in five-spice powders. The leaves are often served as a salad in India or mixed with other vegetables as a side dish. In other countries, like Lebanon or Syria, the baby leaves of the plant serve as seasoning in a special omelet, called an ijjeh, made with flour and onions. In Spain, fennel stems are used to prepare pickled eggplants. In Italy and Germany, fresh fennel leaves are tossed with salad, avocado and chicory, and it serves as a seasoning for fish and egg dishes. The seeds are also one of the main flavorings in Italian sausage.

The Ancient Romans used fennel to improve eye

conditions. They considered it the "herb of sight." In India, the seeds are still chewed raw for this purpose, and the extracts were once mixed in eye tonics to clear cloudy vision. In fact, some animal studies have shown that fennel demonstrates potential in supporting glaucoma.

Historically, fennel juice was made into a syrup to help relieve chronic coughing. It was also used to rid stables and kennels of fleas, as the bugs are driven out by the scent. Additional historical uses for fennel include balancing hormones and stimulating milk production in mothers who are nursing. These uses are associated with fennel's phytoestrogen content, which helps the body regulate estrogen balance, thereby improving the physical, mental, and emotional wellness of women, especially during menstruation or menopause.

Chemical Components

To generate the essential oil from fennel, the seeds must be steam distilled. This results in the oil's key chemical components, which are primarily methyl chavicol, alpha pinene, limonene, cineole, anisic aldehyde, fenchone, myrcene, and trans anethole.

Main Properties of Fennel Essential Oil

Along with the properties previously mentioned in the introduction, fennel oil possesses antioxidant, antispasmodic, antiseptic, antiparasitic, antifungal, antitoxic, diuretic, expectorant, galactogogue, laxative, stimulant, and tonic properties. With such a versatile range, fennel is well equipped to fight off any pathogen in the body's path.

Fennel, as mentioned, is composed of methyl chavicol, alpha pinene, limonene, cineole, anisic aldehyde, fenchone, myrcene, and trans anethole. These components are what instill the enormously beneficial properties within fennel essential oil. We'll outline these properties below.

Antioxidant

Anything high in antioxidants – whether fruit, beans, or essential oils – is a powerful advocate for your body. Antioxidants both protect against free radicals and repair their damage. What are free radicals? Free radicals are destructive chemicals that invade your body, produced by substances both inside and out. Some free radicals (or oxidants) form through normal bodily reactions, like inflammation, metabolism and aerobic respiration. Other free radicals form outside the body, but enter it due to exposure. These include harmful pollutants, toxins, smoking, alcohol, X-rays, and UV rays, to name a few. Although our bodies produce their own antioxidants, these often become damaged as we grow older; thus, introducing antioxidants into our bodies allows these nutrients and enzymes to assist in chemical reactions which destroy the oxidants or free radicals. Fennel essential oil is a moderate antioxidant, aiming to detox the body of free radicals that lead to disease.

Antispasmodic

The antispasmodic properties of fennel oil make it beneficial to such surgical processes as colonoscopy, gastroscopy, and intraluminally-applied double-contrast barium enema.

Antiseptic

The antiseptic and disinfectant properties of fennel essential oil can be reaped topically, applied directly to wounds, or even through burning; the smoke from the oil may help destroy airborne germs. Internal use will help keep the wounds from becoming infections, while external use will support the body's natural function in inhibiting tetanus.

Antiparasitic

Parasites include such mites as fleas, bedbugs, tapeworms, mosquitoes, and lice – pretty much any irritating insect, internal or external, which feeds off the body in one way or another. The human body is a tasty meal to parasites, which can sometimes lead to the transmission of communicable diseases through their feasting off various meals. Fennel is the answer. Its antiparasitic properties will support the body in combating mosquitoes, fleas, bedbugs and lice when applied topically, and intestinal worms when taken orally, which is why fennel is commonly used in insect repellents.

Antifungal

While bacteria and viruses are plenty evil, fungi commonly lead to the deadliest infections, whether external or internal. Your ears, throat and nose are the most likely to become infected by fungi, the infections of which can be both excruciating and unsightly. If left untreated, fungal infections can kill, as they may spread to the brain. Fennel essential oil protects against these infections and more and is particularly effective against skin infections.

Diuretic

If you're looking to lose water weight and reduce blood pressure, fennel essential oil is your agent. The oil stimulates urination, promoting not only the loss of water weight, but the loss of fats, uric acid, sodium, and other body toxins.

Expectorant

Throat or respiratory infections can be staved off and relieved using fennel essential oil. Acting as an expectorant, fennel breaks up and helps destroy the phlegm and mucus buildups that accompany sinuses or respiratory infections. Inflamed throat and lungs – and, thus, coughing – can also be relieved using this oil.

Galactogogue

A galactogogue is a substance that enhances the body's ability to lactate. This can help support mothers who have difficulty producing an enough breast milk for their baby.

Laxative

As a laxative, fennel supplements the body's natural defenses against constipation, by loosening stools and supporting bowel movements.

Stimulant

Stimulants are often referred to as "uppers." This is because they produce mental or physical improvements or temporary enhancements of your bodily functions. For instance, you may grow more alert and awake or quicker on your feet after using a stimulant. Fennel can provide this temporary boost in mental and physical function.

Carminative

By supporting the reduction of excess gas buildup and/or removal of gas from the intestines, fennel essential oil provides relief from abdominal pain, excess sweating, and uncomfortable indigestion.

Emmenagogue

No need to look this one up. An emmenagogue is a menstrual stimulant for those with irregular menses. Fennel regulates hormones, which means that this emmenagogue can also delay and/or reduce the symptoms of menopause, which include hormonal and mood imbalance, nausea, pain, headache, and fatigue.

Stomachic

As a stomachic, fennel improves stomach function, boosts appetite, and helps to tone the stomach. The oil helps control the stomach's bile, acid and gastric liquids.

Tonic

Fennel essential oil benefits each of the body's systems, whether nervous, digestive, respiratory or excretory, making it an unbeatable general tonic. The oil also supports the immune system by helping the body absorb nutrients.

Common Therapeutic Uses

Traditionally used to enhance the body's defenses against digestive conditions, fennel essential oil remains a significant support for gastrointestinal and abdominal issues, protecting against everything from indigestion to diarrhea. Fennel supports cardiovascular wellness, while boosting the immune system and reducing blood pressure. Let's take a closer look at the common uses for this oil.

Cardiovascular Wellness

Cardiovascular wellness can be maintained through the application of fennel essential oil, which contains an exceptional amount of dietary fiber. Fiber, along with the oil's other contents, helps to reduce bad cholesterol (LDL) and boost good cholesterol (HDL), resulting in better cardiovascular wellness. The oil's antioxidant properties and its ability to facilitate the dissolution of cholesterol that accumulates in arteries will also support cardiovascular issues, like heart disease, stroke, or atherosclerosis.

Cancer

Fennel essential oil has shown cytotoxic activity against cancer cell lines. This means fennel is toxic to certain cancer cells, forcing these cells to lose membrane integrity and die rapid deaths through the controlled cell death program called apoptosis. The alkaloid, flavonoid and phenol content in fennel also makes it antitumoral, while the oil demonstrates protective effects against radiation during chemotherapy cancer treatment.

Blood Pressure

As a healthy source of potassium and other nutrients, fennel effectively reduces blood pressure by supporting the relaxation of veins and arteries. This supports overall wellness, as everything in the body – your blood vessels, brain, muscles, and other organs – functions better with increased circulation and oxygenation. Your risks for such issues as stroke, heart attack, brain hemorrhaging, or atherosclerosis are reduced and even your metabolism is given a jolt when blood pressure is optimal. This is also one of the reasons why fennel supports superior cognitive function.

Digestive Wellness

Fennel is a digestive, a carminative, an antispasmodic, a laxative, a tonic, a stomachic, and an emmenagogue and therefore is an effective support when it comes to digestive wellness. Whether you have menstrual cramps, indigestion, nausea, diarrhea, constipation, or upset stomach, a dosage of this oil and its supportive properties will help ease the pain and discomfort of most any stomach issue, while maintaining overall wellness of the gastrointestinal tract.

Immune System Booster

Fennel is a superb immune system support which boosts circulation and increases white blood cell count. The oil's chemical components deliver incredible antifungal, antiparasitic, and antiseptic properties, making it akin to an immune shield braced to fight off angry parasites and fungal strains, like candida. Additionally, the vitamin C content and antioxidant properties fortify the body's system against free radicals and aid general immune function. With such strong armor, this immune stimulant will ensure that your body is better prepared to protect against deadly infections

Women's Wellness

Fennel can benefit women at any age, as it helps balance hormones. Female hormones fluctuate significantly, resulting in the fluctuation of bodily function and emotional and mental wellness. In some cases, this hormonal imbalance can impact their daily lives. Therefore, administering fennel, particularly during periods of menstrual or menopausal influx, can support the body's natural function. If you commonly experience painful or irregular periods or unpleasant menopausal effects, a fennel application will help relieve your menstrual- or menopausal-related condition. The oil is an emmenagogue, meaning it can help young women become regular and relieve painful menstrual cramps, while helping aging women combat unpleasant attributes of menopause, like hot flashes and mood-swings, all by better maintaining hormonal balance. Fennel essential oil also helps regulate other women's issues – lactation, for instance. As a galactogogue, fennel can help support mothers who have difficulty producing enough breast milk for their baby.

Eye Wellness

High in antioxidants, in vitamin C, as well as in minerals like magnesium and cobalt, fennel can protect against macular degeneration and vision conditions. The oil helps reduce the stress placed on our eyes. Fennel leaves contain juice that can relieve eye fatigue or irritation.

Respiratory Issues

As an anti-inflammatory, antiseptic, expectorant, and antifungal, fennel essential oil calms coughing by opening the airways. Bronchitis, congestion, asthma, sinusitis, cough, and other respiratory issues can be supported with fennel essential oil, as the oil's anetol and cineole content promotes a healthy respiratory tract, reduces phlegm, and clears nasal and throat passages.

Safety Precautions & Common Applications

Safety

Certain adverse effects may evolve when using pure essential oils. Some essential oils should not be used when pregnant, for example, as they may cause miscarriage. Allergic reactions, too, may occur, especially when applied topically. Always administer an allergy test before committing fully to topical application. When used with other medications, essential oils may react negatively. If you are on any current prescription medications or have a chronic illness, such as high blood pressure, epilepsy or liver disease, then researching the effects of essential oils against your own personal medical history will eliminate any potentially problematic issues.

Fennel has been approved by the FDA for internal consumption and so can be used as a dietary supplement. Do not use in large quantities, as fennel is a dermal sensitizer. Also avoid or use with caution if pregnant or epileptic. If you have sensitive skin, dilute heavily and test before extensive use. Otherwise, the oil can be used neat or undiluted. You can apply topically, diffuse or use as a dietary supplement.

Blends

Oftentimes, essential oils are manufactured as blends of several pure oils. For instance, the Protective Blend of certain brands is a mix of cinnamon, clove, rosemary, and eucalyptus. This blend can be used to boost the immune system to help support colds, viruses and flus. The downside to blends is that the more oils added to the mix, the higher the probability your patient may react negatively to the blend if he/she is prone to allergies. There is also the possibility of phototoxicity when working with blends, particularly if they include citrus oils. Be sure to read your labels before administering.

Regardless of these possible effects, essential oils are a viable option for supporting several conditions. Those looking to support or maintain their own personal wellness, or that of their families', should become educated on the uses of essential oils, their natural remedies and the methods of application. Only then can you begin building your kit of essential oils for survival.

Chapter 2 – Recipes for Fennel Essential Oil

In this chapter, we'll offer various recipes for fennel essential oil, both for pure fennel applications and blends. For pure applications, we've provided the appropriate dosage and method of administration to support specific ailments, from blood clots to stomach cramps. When it comes to blends, herbalists and aromatherapists often combine fennel essential oil with geranium, sandalwood, lavender, and rose. We'll offer some fantastic blending options in the second half of this chapter.

Pure Applications

Anxiety

When you're feeling overwhelmed, calm yourself by placing a drop of fennel essential oil into your hands, rubbing your palms together, cupping them over your nose, and breathing deeply in and out for several minutes.

Blood Clots

To support the body's natural defenses against blood clots, topically apply fennel essential oil, either neat or diluted in a 1:1 ratio with a carrier oil, over the area of concern. You can also diffuse or take internally by adding a drop to a glass of water. *Ask your doctor to support this application before use.

Bruises

Accelerate the support process when it comes to bruising by applying 1-2 drops of fennel essential oil, either neat or diluted in a 1:1 ratio with a carrier oil, over the affected area.

Courage

To enhance courage or bravery, place a drop of fennel essential oil into your hands, rub your palms together, cup them over your nose, and breathe deeply in and out for several minutes. You can also diffuse throughout your home or apply topically, using either neat or in a 1:1 dilution ratio, and massaging into the solar plexus. Apply daily for the best results.

Detoxing

Support the body's systems through detoxification by using neat or combining fennel essential oil in a 1:1 ratio with a carrier oil and massaging toward the heart. You can also place 1 drop to a glass of drinking water and take internally.

Digestive Aid

Fennel aids the digestive tract and can be taken orally or applied topically. Place a drop into your drinking water for internal consumption, or dilute the oil in a 1:3 ratio with a carrier oil and apply topically to the abdomen in a clockwise motion and into the reflex points of the feet. You can also diffuse throughout the home.

Flatulence

Relieve gas by using neat or diluting fennel essential oil in a 1:1 ratio with a carrier oil and massaging into the abdomen in a clockwise motion. You can also place a drop in a glass of water and take orally.

Gastritis

Support the body's defenses against gastritis by placing a drop of fennel essential oil into your drinking water and consuming daily.

Hormone Balance

Regulate hormonal balance by using neat or diluting fennel in a 1:1 ratio with a carrier oil and massaging into the reflex points of the feet. You can also inhale directly from the bottle every day to help maintain balance.

Intestinal Parasite

Rid of intestinal parasites by using neat or diluting fennel essential oil in a 1:1 ratio with a carrier oil and massaging it into the abdomen and the soles of the feet. You can also add a drop to your drinking water.

Kidney Stones

Support the body's natural defenses against kidney stone issues by using fennel essential oil neat or diluting it in a 1:1 ratio with a carrier oil; then apply topically, massaging it over the affected area, three times daily.

Lactation (Increase)

Increase lactation by using neat or diluting fennel essential oil in a 1:1 ratio with a carrier oil; then apply topically, massaging into the breasts toward the lymph nodes (underarms) twice daily. Avoid using more than 10 days.

Liver Support

Support liver function by using neat or diluting fennel

essential oil in a 1:1 ratio with a carrier oil; then apply topically, massaging over the affected area and into the reflex points of the feet. You can also place a drop in your drinking water and take internally daily.

Menstrual Cramps

Alleviate menstrual cramps by using neat or diluting fennel essential oil in a 1:1 ratio with a carrier oil and applying topically. Massage into the lower abdomen and back and into the reflex points of the feet.

Motivation

Give yourself a motivational boost by diffusing throughout your home or car. You can also place a drop on your shirt sleeve or inhale directly whenever you're feeling stressed.

Nausea

Stave off or relieve nausea by applying a single drop to a piece of cloth or on the shirt collar to be inhaled when feeling nauseous. You can also diffuse or apply fennel essential oil neat or diluted in a 1:1 ratio with a carrier oil, massaging the solution into the abdomen. You can also take internally. Place a drop in your drinking water and drink slowly.

Pancreas Support

Fennel helps regulate blood sugar and promotes pancreas function. Use neat or diluted in a 1:1 ratio with a carrier oil and apply topically over the pancreas or massage into the soles of the feet. You might also use it as a dietary supplement or add a drop to each meal.

PMS

Relieve PMS symptoms by diffusing throughout your cycle. You can also use neat or dilute fennel essential oil in a 1:1 ratio with a carrier oil and massage it into the reflex points of the feet on a regular basis throughout the month.

Prostate Support

To support the prostate, use neat or dilute fennel essential oil in a 1:1 ratio with a carrier oil and apply it over the area of concern and into the reflex points of the feet on a regular basis.

Prostatic Hyperplasia (Benign Enlargement of the Prostate)

Use the same application as above. You might also add a drop to your drinking water and take internally every day.

Skin Renewal

Renew and revitalize the skin by placing a drop of fennel essential oil into your moisturizer or cleanser each time you follow your skin regimen.

Stomach Cramps

Alleviate menstrual cramps by using neat or diluting fennel essential oil in a 1:1 ratio with a carrier oil and applying topically. Massage into the lower abdomen and back and into the reflex points of the feet.

Strength

Promote strength within by placing a drop of fennel essential oil into your hands, rubbing your palms together, cupping them over your nose, and breathing deeply in and out for several minutes.

Urinary Stones

Support the body's natural defenses against urinary stone issues by using fennel essential oil neat or diluting it in a 1:1 ratio with a carrier oil; then apply topically, massaging it over the affected area. You can also place a drop in your drinking water and take internally.

Wrinkles

Protect against wrinkles by adding a drop of fennel essential oil to your moisturizer and massaging it into the affected area. Be careful around the eyes.

Blends

Anti-Wrinkle Solution

Ingredients

- 2 drops Rosemary Essential Oil
- 3 drops Lemon Essential Oil
- 10 drops Lavender Essential Oil
- 10 drops Fennel Essential Oil
- 10 drops Neroli Essential Oil
- 10 drops Frankincense Essential Oil
- 10 drops Carrot Essential Oil
- 10 drops Primrose Essential Oil
- 2 Tbsps. Sweet Almond Oil

Directions

To protect against and reduce the appearance of wrinkles, place all ingredients into a small glass bowl or container and mix well. Apply to the neck and face before bed each night, massaging into problem areas in a circular motion.

Constipation/Diarrhea

Ingredients

- 2 drops Fennel Essential Oil
- 2 drops Peppermint Essential Oil
- 1 drop Ginger Essential Oil

Directions

To relieve constipation or diarrhea, place all ingredients into a "00" capsule and ingest every three hours until the issue is resolved.

Courage Blend

Ingredients

- 3 drops Thyme Essential Oil
- 2 drops Fennel Essential Oil
- 1 drop Black Pepper Essential Oil
- 1 drop Ginger Essential Oil
- ½ cup Epsom Salt

Directions

To combat negative thoughts and stimulate courage, add all ingredients to your bathwater and stir to disperse. Then inhale deeply while you soak for 20 minutes, but avoid getting water in your eyes, as it may sting.

Craving Crasher

Ingredients

- 6 drops Fennel Essential Oil
- 3 drops Ginger Essential Oil
- 2 drops Rosemary Essential Oil
- 1 drop Black Pepper Essential Oil

Directions

Enhance your weight-loss by placing all ingredients into a small glass bottle or container. Inhale several times an hour to suppress appetite or combat cravings.

Diuretic Bath

Ingredients

- 3 drops Juniper Essential Oil
- 3 drops Lemon Essential Oil
- 2 drops Fennel Essential Oil

Directions

Support bodily detoxification by place all ingredients into your bathwater and stirring to disperse. Then inhale deeply while you soak for 20 minutes, but avoid getting water in your eyes, as it may sting.

Gout

Ingredients

- 6 drops Lemon Essential Oil
- 6 drops Juniper Essential Oil
- 3 drops Fennel Essential Oil
- 25 mL Grapeseed Oil

Directions

To relieve gout, combine all ingredients in a bowl or container and blend well. Massage over the affected area.

Hot Flash Relief

Ingredients

- 1 drop Fennel Essential Oil
- 1 drop Palmarosa Essential Oil
- 1 drop Clary Sage Essential Oil
- 3 drops Carrier Oil

Directions

Relieve hot flashes by combining all ingredients in a small glass container and applying topically to your pulse points.

Indigestion

Ingredients

- 3 drops Fennel Essential Oil
- 3 drops Sage Essential Oil
- 5 drops Orange Essential Oil

Directions

To relieve indigestion, combine all ingredients into a small bowl or container and blend well. Apply topically over the chest and back, massaging into the affected area. Do not use immediately following a meal, as massaging can interfere with digestion.

Lymphatic Support

Ingredients

- 2 drops Geranium Essential Oil
- 2 drops Rosemary Essential Oil
- 3 drops Clary Sage Essential Oil
- 6 drops Fennel Essential Oil
- 25 mL Grapeseed Oil

Directions

To enhance lymphatic drainage of tissues, place all ingredients in a small bowl or jar and blend well. Apply topically, massaging into the lymph nodes.

Regulate Menstruation

Ingredients

- 2 drops Fennel Essential Oil
- 2 drops Basil Essential Oil
- 2 drops Melissa Essential Oil

Directions

Support menstrual wellness and help regulate periods by placing the oils in a large bowl of hot water. Make a hot compress by soaking a hand towel or flannel rag in the water. Ring out the excess water and place the compress over the abdomen.

Reproductive Wellness Salve

Ingredients

- 4 drops Fennel Essential Oil
- 4 drops Clary Sage Essential Oil
- 4 drops Cypress Essential Oil
- 30 mL Sweet Almond Oil

Directions

Support reproductive wellness by placing all ingredients in a small glass bowl or container and mixing thoroughly, then apply the salve to the back and stomach regularly.

Stomach Cramps

Ingredients

- 6 drops Rosemary Essential Oil
- 3 drops Fennel Essential Oil
- 1 drop Peppermint Essential Oil

Directions

To relieve cramps, place all ingredients into a bowl of hot water and blend well. Soak a towel or piece of flannel in the water to make a hot compress. Place across the stomach.

Stress-Reducing Massage Oil

Ingredients

- 1 Tbsp. Carrier Oil
- 1 drop Lavender Essential Oil
- 3 drops Cinnamon Bark Essential Oil
- 3 drops Grapefruit Essential Oil
- 4 drops Fennel Essential Oil
- 4 drops Roman Chamomile Essential Oil
- 5 drops Melissa Essential Oil

Directions

In a small bowl or jar, combine oils, mixing until evenly distributed. Massage the oil into the shoulders, back and neck. Recommended for two-time use before a stressful event, 6 hours apart to help relieve anxiety.

Swollen Feet

Ingredients

- 5 drops Fennel Essential Oil
- 5 drops Cypress Essential Oil
- 20 mL Grapeseed Oil

Directions

To relieve swollen feet, especially during pregnancy, place all ingredients in a small glass bowl or container and mixing thoroughly, then apply the salve to ankles and feet.

Uplifting Blend

Ingredients

- 3 drops Fennel Essential Oil
- 3 drops Marjoram Essential Oil
- 4 drop Lemon Essential Oil

Directions

To uplift the spirit, place all ingredients into your vaporizer and use as normal.

Water Retention

Ingredients

- 2 drops Peppermint Essential Oil
- 3 drops Fennel Essential Oil
- 5 drop Juniper Essential Oil
- 10 drops Lemon Essential Oil
- 25 mL Sweet Almond Oil

Directions

To combat bloating, combine all ingredients in a small bowl or jar and blend well. Apply topically, massaging into the lower back and abdomen.

Chapter 3 – Fennel Essential Oil Studies

Many studies have been done on essential oils to uncover and prove their therapeutic qualities. In the case of the great number of fennel studies, many of the properties attributed to the essential oil (noted in this book and elsewhere) are quite often validated through the research from accredited universities and published by reputable scientific journals. In this chapter, we'll discuss a small portion of these studies. It's important to note that research on essential oils is constantly evolving. Keep up with any recent research, as it may turn up even further valuable uses for these miracle oils.

Study 1 – Anxiolytic Activity

In this study published in *BMC Complementary & Alternative Medicine*, the anxiolytic activity of fennel essential oil on was examined, with the following results: "The objective of study was to evaluate the anxiolytic activity of the essential oil of Foeniculum vulgare Miller...The essential oil of F. vulgare was found to exhibit a promising anxiolytic activity."

To study the anxiolytic effect of Foeniculum vulgare, mice were randomly divided into six groups, with the first and second groups receiving Tween 80 (5%, v/v) and diazepam (0.5 mg/kg, ip), respectively, while the third and fourth groups received varying dosages from 50-400 mg/kg of fennel essential oil. The mice were then tested in animal-anxiety models to evaluate the effects. The results showed that the essential oil groups fared better than the control groups, which indicates that fennel essential oil can be used to support anxiety.

Reference
http://www.ncbi.nlm.nih.gov/pubmed/25149087

http://www.ncbi.nlm.nih.gov/pmc/articles/PMC4156641/

Study 2 – Antimicrobial Properties

In this study available on PubMed, the antimicrobial properties of fennel essential oil were examined, with the following results: "In this study the composition and antimicrobial properties of essential oils obtained from Origanum onites, Mentha piperita, Juniperus exalsa, Chrysanthemum indicum, Lavandula hybrida, Rosa damascena, Echinophora tenuifolia, Foeniculum vulgare were examined... Escherichia coli (ATTC 25922), Staphylococcus aureus (ATCC 25923) and Pseudomonas aeruginosa (ATTC 27853) were used as standard test bacterial strains…We also examined the in vitro antimicrobial activities of some components of the essential oils and found some components with antimicrobial activity."

The study examined the antibacterial and antimicrobial activities of eight essential oil extracts – including fennel essential oil – against Staphylococcus aureus, Pseudomonas aeruginosa, and Escherichia coli.

Staphylococcus aureus is a Gram-positive bacterium. Although Staphylococcus aureus is part of the normal human skin flora and respiratory tract and is not typically pathogenic, those with compromised immune systems can potentially develop an infection from the bacteria. When it becomes pathogenic, S. aureus produces respiratory issues like sinusitis, skin infections, and even food poisoning.

Pseudomonas aeruginosa is also a common bacteria

found in water, soil, skin flora, and in man-made environments. The bacterium thrives on moist surfaces, and so can threaten the hospital environment by finding its home on medical equipment, like catheters, resulting in cross-infection. It is, for instance, the bacterium which causes hot-tub rash. This bacterium also attacks immunocompromised patients, infecting the urinary tract, airway, wounds, burns, and resulting in blood infections.

Escherichia coli is a bacterium, as well, though it's Gram negative, rather than Gram positive, like S. aureus. E. coli can often result in serious food poisoning.

The study showed that some components of fennel essential oil demonstrated antimicrobial activity against the bacteria tested.

Reference
http://www.ncbi.nlm.nih.gov/pubmed/12510839]

Study 3 – Antioxidant, Anti-inflammatory & Anti-proliferative Properties

In this study available on PubMed, the antioxidant, anti-inflammatory and anti-proliferative activities of fennel essential oil were examined, with the following results: "Essential oils (EO) possess antimicrobial, anti-inflammatory, insect repellent, anti-cancer, and antioxidant properties, among others. In the present work, the antioxidant, anti-inflammatory and anti-proliferative activities of Moroccan commercial EOs (Citrus aurantium, C. limon, Cupressus sempervirens, Eucalyptus globulus, Foeniculum vulgare and Thymus vulgaris) were evaluated and compared with their main constituents....T. vulgaris EO showed the best free radicals scavenging capacity. This EO was also the most effective against lipid peroxidation along with C. limon and F. vulgare EOs...The antioxidant and anti-inflammatory activities of the EOs were plant species dependent and not always attributable to the EOs main components. Nevertheless, the EOs anti-proliferative activities were more related to their main components, as with T. vulgaris, C. limon, E. globulus and C. sempervirens."

This study examined Citrus aurantium, Citrus limon, Cupressus sempervirens, Eucalyptus globulus, Foeniculum vulgare and Thymus vulgaris essential oils. The objective was to compare the essential oils' antioxidant, anti-inflammatory and anti-proliferative activities with that of their main components. The study found that all oils demonstrated antioxidant, anti-inflammatory and anti-proliferative activities, but that the antioxidant and anti-inflammatory activities of the oils were not always directly attributed to the oils' main components, while the anti-proliferative activities were. This likely indicates that the antioxidant and anti-inflammatory activities of fennel are the result of the synergistic effect of all the oil's components, while its main components are responsible for the oil's anti-proliferative activities. Fennel essential oil was also one of the most effective against lipid peroxidation.

Reference

http://www.ncbi.nlm.nih.gov/pubmed/24868891]

Study 4 – Antifungal Properties

In this study available on PubMed, the antifungal effects of fennel essential oil were examined, with the following results: "Fennel seed essential oil (FSEO) is a plant-derived natural therapeutic against dermatophytes. In this study, the antifungal effects of FSEO were investigated from varied aspects...The results indicated that FSEO had potent antifungal activities on Trichophyton rubrum ATCC 40051, Trichophyton tonsurans 10-0400, Microsporum gypseum 44693-1 and Trichophyton mentagrophytes 10-0060, which is better than the commonly used antifungal agents fluconazole and amphotericin B...With better antifungal activity than the commonly used antifungal agents and less possibility of inducing drug resistance, FSEO could be used as a potential antidermatophytic agent."

This study tested fennel essential oil against several fungi – including Trichophyton rubrum, Trichophyton tonsurans, Microsporum gypseum, and Trichophyton mentagrophytes. Trichophyton rubrum is a dermatophytic fungus that colonizes the dead skin in the upper layers, which can cause nail fungal infections, athlete's foot, ringworm, and jock itch. Trichophyton tonsurans is a fungus that can cause ringworm infection in the scalp. Microsporum gypseum is a dermatophyte that's associated with soil and infects the dead skin in upper layers, causing fungal infections of the skin. Trichophyton interdigitale is one of three regular fungi to cause ringworm in animals and tinea infections in humans. It also causes zoonotic skin disease, which is when mycotic skin disease is transferred from human to animal or vice versa. The fungus is found most often in rodents, but also in rabbits, horses, and dogs.

Fennel essential oil was effective against these fungi. In fact, the antifungal mechanism of the oil was to destroy the plasma membrane and intracellular organelles, while inhibiting the mitochondrial enzyme activities. The study demonstrated that fennel essential oil is an effective antifungal.

Reference
http://www.ncbi.nlm.nih.gov/pubmed/25351709]

Study 5 – Antifungal Properties

In this study published in the *Asian Pacific Journal of Biomedicine*, the antifungal effects of fennel essential oil were examined, with the following results: "To investigate effect of essential oils on Aspergillus spore germination, growth and mycotoxin production…in vitro antifungal and antiaflatoxigenic activity of essential oils was carried out using poisoned food techniques, spore germination assay, agar dilution assay, and aflatoxin arresting assay on toxigenic strains of Aspergillus species… Cymbopogon martinii, Foeniculum vulgare and T. ammi oils as antifungal were found superior over synthetic preservative. In conclusion, the essential oils…can be a potential source of safe natural food preservative for food commodities contamination by storage fungi."

This study investigated fennel essential oil's antifungal activity against several Aspergillus species, including Aspergillus niger and Aspergillus flavus. Aspergillus niger is a fungus that causes black mold disease on some fruits and vegetables, like onions, apricots, grapes, and peanuts. A.niger is a common food contaminant, thrives in soil, and grows in indoor environments as well, which can cause wellness problems for inhabitants. Aspergillus flavus is a pathogenic fungus appearing in cereal grains, tree nuts, and legumes, during stages of harvest, transit, or storage. Many Aspergillus flavus strains produce toxic compounds, called mycotoxins, which are toxic when consumed. A. flavus can also produce opportunistic human pathogens, causing aspergillosis, which may result in tuberculosis or ear, eye, nose, or nail infection in immunocompromised individuals.

All three of the essential oils tested were shown to possess superior antifungal properties over the synthetic preservative. This demonstrates the potential for use of these essential oils as food preservatives to protect against contamination by these strains of fungi.

Reference
http://www.ncbi.nlm.nih.gov/pubmed/25183114

http://www.ncbi.nlm.nih.gov/pmc/articles/PMC4025292/pdf/apjtb-04-s1-s373.pdf

Study 6 – Anticarcinogenic & Antioxidant Properties

In this study published by the *Journal of Medical Food*, the anticarcinogenic and antioxidant properties of fennel essential oil were examined, with the following results: "The present study evaluated the efficacy of fennel seed methanolic extract (FSME) for its antioxidant, cytotoxic, and antitumor activities and for its capacity to serve as a nontoxic radioprotector in Swiss albino mice. We also assessed the natural antioxidant compounds of FSME for use in industrial application...FSME also exhibited an antitumor effect by modulating lipid peroxidation and augmenting the antioxidant defense system in EAC-bearing mice with or without exposure to radiation."

The cytotoxicity of fennel essential oil was tested on mice injected with breast cancer cells and liver cells. Fennel demonstrated remarkable anticancer potential against liver cancer cell and breast cancer cell lines. The oil also demonstrated strong free radical-scavenging activity, indicating that fennel is high in antioxidants. These results suggest the potential efficacy for use of fennel essential oil in supporting the body's defenses against liver and breast cancers, as well as reducing oxidative stress.

Reference
http://www.ncbi.nlm.nih.gov/pubmed/21812646]

Chapter 4 – The Ins & Outs of Essential Oils

Where do essential oils come from?

Plants and plant species naturally produce essential oils for various reasons, one being to draw pollinator insects to them, another being to repel invading organisms (bacteria, animals). Several chemical compounds compose each plant's essential oil, and the combination of these compounds are specific to each oil, which then instills in the oil its own unique properties. Essential oils can be harnessed from all sorts of plant components, including flowers, leaves, bark, fruit, roots, and resin. For instance, cinnamon oil is harnessed from bark, lemon oil from the peel, and lavender oil from lavender flowers. Certain plants can produce a few chemical variants of the same essential oil, which are acquired from different parts of the plant.

Some of these parts produce a large amount of oil, while others produce just a smidgen. The oil's quality and potency depends upon several factors, including the subspecies of the plant, its soil conditions, the time of year and even the time of day you harvest it.

How are essential oils extracted?

Essential oils can be extracted from plants through various methods, including pressing, distillation, solvent and maceration. Let's take a brief look at each:

Pressing Method

Commonly used with citrus fruit, the pressing method extracts the oil through a technique which involves pushing the fruit peels through a press. Oily fruits and plants are best suited for this technique. Orange oil, for example, is extracted from orange skins through the pressing method.

Distillation Method

This technique harkens back to the days of old-timey moonshiners, as the same sort of method used to create strong liquor can be used to extract essential oils. Using a still, boiled water and plant materials will create steam which is then cooled by coils and condensed into a combination of water and oil. This combination doesn't mix, so the oil can then be extracted from it.

Solvent Method

Through a multi-step process, certain plant and flower oils can be extracted using alcohol and other solvents, which extort the essential oil from the plant materials.

Maceration Method

When a "carrier" or fixed oil or lard is mixed with the plant material and set out in the sun, over a period, the carrier oil is infused with the plant's essence. Heat sources, other than the sun, are often used to speed the process. Throughout the process, more plant material is added to produce a more potent oil.

How do you use essential oils?

Although some studies about the effectiveness of essential oils are conducted by small companies or even individuals, several them are conducted by the food and cosmetic industries. In general, the pharmaceutical industry shows next to no interest in herbal medicine, primarily because there are few options to patent such products. Being as such, the product's lack of profitability results in a lack of research funding. Regardless, the historical uses of essential oils tell us what we need to know: these oils have been effectively administered for centuries. The therapeutic qualifications of essential oils can be plotted in the survival of humans across cultures and generations.

Another reason that studies on essential oils have not resulted in much conclusive evidence as to their overall effectiveness is because definitive results are sometimes difficult to prove, as the quality of each batch of oil can vary for several reasons. One is that essential oils are impossible to standardize. As mentioned above, even the slightest variance in soil conditions and the time of harvesting – as well as innumerable other factors – will produce a different product quality and potency. In addition, essential oils are often obtained from various species of the same plant; Eucalyptus radiata and Eucalyptus globulus can both be used in the making of therapeutic-grade eucalyptus oil and, as a result, they may have slightly different properties and degrees of strength or effectiveness.

Just as there are several methods by which to extract essential oils, there are several methods to administer them therapeutically. The variety of chemical compounds in each essential oil means that their benefits and applications also vary across the board. Below are a few of these methods.

Topical Administration

Direct application of many essential oils works like a sponge, as skin sops up chemicals and other things (like sunlight, for instance). Topical application is best when you want to clear up an ailment on the skin's surface or in the underlying muscle tissue. When applying topically, you may either massage the oil into the skin or simply dab on the skin for therapeutic results. You might combine the essential oil with a carrier oil for topical use to dilute its potency. This is safer, as the oil is so concentrated. You may support your body's defenses against rash or muscle pain in this manner, but you should always test your patient for allergens before applying. Adverse effects are produced by natural chemicals as much as synthetic ones; poison ivy, for example.

To test for allergens, place a drop or two on your patient's inner forearm. If a rash develops within 12 to 24 hours, then the patient is allergic. In addition, phototoxicity – sun exposure resulting in an exacerbated burn – may be an issue when citrus oils are applied topically. So, one must proceed with caution when applying essential oils using this method.

Inhalation Therapy

Commonly known as "aromatherapy", this essential oil application is effective for inner ailments, like sore throat or cold. In a steaming bowl of distilled or sterilized water, add a few drops of essential oil and, with a towel over your head, bend over the bowl and inhale. The towel captures the vapors, making the technique even more effective. Essential oils can also be placed in a diffuser or potpourri throughout a room to produce somewhat diluted medicinal effects.

Ingestion

When using this method, proceed with caution. Direct ingestion of essential oils must be monitored and applied in small doses that are diluted in a tablespoon or more of any carrier oil – olive oil, for example. If you are unsure of dosage amounts, make a tea with the relevant herb instead. Although the effects of this diluted use may be weaker, this application is a better alternative than an overdose of essential oils.

What are the general benefits of using essential oils?

Replacement for Prescription Drugs

One practical benefit for using essential oils is, of course, their substitutive nature. Many believe that they can replace Rx drugs, which is the ultimate reason to educate yourself on their application and to begin stockpiling your essential oil supply. Although it is our opinion that 100% pure essential oils that carry no harmful side effects are better to support the body and its functions, we recommend that you consult your physician before replacing your prescription or over-the-counter medications.

One of the potential threats of economic or social collapse is the lack of resources, and primarily the inability to procure prescription drugs. Being as such, finding suitable alternatives should be a priority when prepping for the worst.

Their portability is also a major bonus when it comes to survival prepping. The fact that these ultra-concentrated oils take up little-to-no space makes toting them to your shelter all the simpler should the need arise. And, because essential oils are highly concentrated, the application used in most procedures requires only a drop or two of oil, which means that tiny bottle will be long-lasting (example 15mL bottle contains approx. 250 drops).

Cheap, but Effective Alternative

Though money may be the last thing on your mind when it comes to prepping for a survival situation (money may even be obsolete in the event of social collapse), it is worth noting that the expense of essential oils pales in comparison to prescription drugs. In fact, whether you are forced to survive on essential oils due to a lack of prescription reserves, in some cases, you might consider substituting your prescriptions for these inexpensive alternatives regardless. Essential oils are a cheap, but equally effective alternative to prescription medicine.

No Expiration Date

Another benefit of essential oils is that they do not expire, neither do they have "proper storage" requirements. Several medicines and therapeutic products must be replaced every couple years, so this sets essential oils ahead of the pack when it comes to shelf life.

Versatility

Essential oils also offer great versatility. Apart from providing wellness benefits, essential oils can be repurposed for household and hygienic applications. For instance, if you're looking for something that might serve your dental hygiene needs in a time of crisis, thieves oil is your go-to essential oil. If you want to maintain your skin's wellness, frankincense and lavender will do the trick; the latter also serves as sunscreen, so you can prevent sun damage as well.

When it comes to the house or shelter, you can use essential oils to deodorize, which will come in handy in a disaster scenario where things might start to smell fishy due to lack of proper utilities and care. For example, after the 2011 tsunami and the subsequent nuclear reactor meltdown in Japan, a nurse named Risa Nakahira used essential oils to deodorize and sanitize putrid public bathrooms in overpopulated evacuation facilities. As relief workers searched for survivors, often wading through debris and decay, Nakahira also deodorized their boots and masks using essential oils. The possibilities of these natural oils are endless.

They are also versatile when it comes to the range of patients they're capable of supporting. The wellness of everyone from your great grandfather to your infant baby can be fortified with the aid of essential oils in the appropriate dosage. They even come in handy when supporting the wellness of livestock or pets. From teething infants to dementia in the elderly, from teenagers with acne to dogs with urinary tract infections, essential oils can serve any patient with nearly any ailment.

Conclusion

Now that you know all about what fennel essential oil can do for you – where it originates, how it's extracted, its benefits and properties, and the different methods of administration – you can use it confidently to support the body's defenses against wellness issues and start to assemble a kit of essential oils for survival.

The various benefits of essential oils and their properties are countless. To build your own kit, first focus on acquiring the essential oils which may bear more relevance to your wellness issues or the potential wellness threats within your environment. When it comes to women's wellness, for instance, fennel essential oil will be one of your more crucial oils, due to its hormonal balancing and feminine supportive properties.

Used as a supplement or as your go-to for menopausal and menstrual issues, cardiovascular function, or digestive wellness, the application of fennel essential oil in medicine has survived for centuries and will survive centuries more. When it comes down to it, you don't need to rely on pharmaceuticals; essential oils, herbs, and plenty of other natural ingredients can be used to help support any number of wellness issues, whether ailment or injury.

Essential oils are essential to your survival in the case of viral outbreak, social collapse or natural disaster because, when the SHTF, your access to pharmaceuticals will likely either be limited or eliminated altogether. Alternatives to our modern-day standard will equate survival when no other option exists. And when it comes to a life-or-death situation, you can't let your wellness decline, no matter the state of the world.

DISCLAIMER AND/OR LEGAL NOTICES: Every effort has been made to accurately represent this book and it's potential. Results vary with every individual, and your results may or may not be different from those depicted. No promises, guarantees or warranties, whether stated or implied, have been made that you will produce any specific result from this book. Your efforts are individual and unique, and may vary from those shown. Your success depends on your efforts, background and motivation.

The material in this publication is provided for educational and informational purposes only and is not intended as medical advice. The information contained in this book should not be used to diagnose or treat any illness, metabolic disorder, disease or health problem. Always consult your physician or healthcare provider before beginning any nutrition or exercise program. Use of the programs, advice, and information contained in this book is at the sole choice and risk of the reader.